Natural Support for Babies being Vaccinated

Using Homeopathy, Tissue Salts & Other Natural Remedies

An overview of natural alternatives to vaccinations plus a step by step guide on how to use Homeopathy, Tissue Salts, Bach Flowers & other Natural Remedies to gently support & detox baby if you do choose to vaccinate or partially vaccinate.

by Dorae Smith
LLB, ND, Dip Hom

Text copyright © Dorae Smith
2018
Copyright © bubiroo books

Cover Design by Dorae Smith
Cover Image copyright © Dorae Smith

Contact details: bubiroo@gmail.com
2018

ISBN: 9781717800572

All rights reserved. No part of this publication may be reproduced, stored in a retrieval system, or transmitted, in any form or by any means, electronic, mechanical, photocopying, recording or otherwise without the prior permission of the publishers.

This book contains a selection of natural remedies that may be considered as an alternative to vaccinations and more importantly remedies that may be useful in supporting babies before and after vaccination. It is intended as an aid to learning about and understanding their use. It is not intended to replace or supersede consultation with, or treatment from, a qualified professional. The book does not represent an endorsement or guarantee as to the appropriateness or efficacy of a remedy.

Contents

INTRODUCTION 4
   What is Homeopathy? 4
      Selecting the Appropriate Remedy 5
      Potency and Dosage 5
   What are Biochemical Tissues Salts? 6
      Potency and Dosage 6
   What are Bach Flower Remedies? 7
      Dosage 7
HOMEOPROPHYLAXIS – 8
A NATURAL ALTERNATIVE TO VACCINATION 8
   The Isaac Golden Homoeoprophylaxis Program 9
   Prophylactic Remedies 10
   Supplementary Protection Program 11
SIDE-EFFECTS OF VACCINATIONS 14
   Potential Short-term Side-effects 14
   Potential Long-term Side-effects 14
MINIMISING VACCINATION SIDE-EFFECTS 16
   Mental and Emotional Support 16
   Physical Support 16
   Holistic Support using Homeopathy 17
   Isopathic Treatment 18
VACCINATION DETOX PROGRAMS 20
   Homeopathic Vaccination Detox 20
   Tissue Salt Vaccination Detox 21
   Detox Bath 21
   Vaccination Support Kit Shopping List 22
BIBLIOGRAPHY 23
ABOUT THE AUTHOR 24

INTRODUCTION

Choosing to vaccinate one's baby or not has become such a contentious subject that it will most probably be one of the first topics that come up in conversation when you announce you're expecting.

Once baby is here, the question of whether you vaccinate or not will almost always come up. And very often, depending on the company you find yourself IN, you're damned if you do and damned if you don't. There are two very defined camps with seemingly little space for compromise. You're expected to be either 100% pro-vaccinating or 100% anti-vaccinating.

That said, it is a very personal choice! And for many it is also a very difficult choice to make. There is a wealth of information available to enable one to make an informed choice. Which is why this booklet will only touch on the subject very briefly. It will outline Natural Alternatives to vaccinating but focus on what can be done to support baby if you decide to vaccinate or partially vaccinate.

Homeopathy in particular can be very useful in making the process less traumatic, reducing the risks associated with vaccinating and also easing the discomfort which my follow immunisations.

The remedies are perfectly safe as well as non-addictive and carry no risk of toxicity or side effects. The same applies to Biochemical Tissue Salts as well as Bach Flower Remedies.

What is Homeopathy?

Homeopathy is a science of healing created in the 18th century by Dr Samuel Hahnemann, a German physician and chemist. It is based on the law of similars. In other words, it works on the principal that like cures like. A simplified example would be that a remedy such as Arnica works wonders for bruising when given in homeopathic form. If you were to take the crude form in high doses it would in fact cause bruising.

Constitutional prescribing treats the individual as a whole. The appropriate remedy is selected by taking into account emotional, physical, spiritual and mental signs, characteristics and idiosyncrasies as well as responses to everyday and life-changing events. The remedy will work on a very deep level to strengthen the body and encourage the vital force to deal with the root cause of the problem. The body is then able to heal itself.

The remedies suggested in this book are for use as part of a protocol. It is NOT constitutional treatment but rather it is akin to First Aid prescribing.

Furthermore, where a remedy is expanded upon, there is always a lot more to be said for each remedy. However, for the purposes of this book only a very concise description of the remedy picture is given, and only insofar as it applies to vaccinations and their side-effects.

Homeopathic remedies are perfectly safe to be used during pregnancy and on newborn babies and can be taken alongside other medication.

Selecting the Appropriate Remedy

Most of the remedies indicated in this guide form part of the Homeoprophylaxis Program, Pre- and Post-Vaccination Protocols and Detox Programs. You are therefore not required to select any remedies unless you are treating an acute illness such as Chicken Pox, Measles etc. You simply use the remedies noted in the manner explained.

Using homeopathy in your daily life for first aid or as home remedies e.g. to minimise a bout of flu or mumps will be different. When deciding on the remedy that is needed in such instances please remember that not all the symptoms mentioned in a materia medica need to be present. What you are looking for is the remedy picture that includes all or most of the symptoms being felt.

Potency and Dosage

Once again, because we are focused on protocols and programs you simply need to administer the remedies in the potency indicated and as described.

If you were to use the remedies for first aid or general home remedies during acute ailments, then the process is different. A general guideline would be:

Take the remedy, and then wait.
If an improvement is felt, take nothing until the symptoms return.
Then either

- repeat the remedy or
- if the symptom picture has changed, take a different remedy as indicated.

Homeopathic remedies are taken by simply placing the pillules under the tongue and allowing them to dissolve. Alternatively, they can be added to water, allowed to dissolve and the water sipped.

The remedy should be taken on a clean palette. Food, drinks and even brushing teeth should be avoided for 20 minutes before and after taking the remedy.

What are Biochemical Tissues Salts?

Dr Wilhelm Schussler researched the most common mineral tissue salts found in the human body. Based on his findings he identified 12 minerals that he believed to be vital to human health.

Biochemical Tissue or Cell Salts are these 12 minerals prepared in such a way that they are halfway between a nutritional supplement and a homeopathic remedy. As a result, they still contain minute quantities of the original substances.

Tissue Salts work by gradually correcting imbalances or deficiencies of minerals in the body.

They are perfectly safe even for newborn babies and can be taken alongside other medication.

Potency and Dosage

Tissue Salts come in only one potency, 6x. In some countries this potency is denoted as D6.

Tissue Salts are taken by simply placing the pillules under the tongue and allowing them to dissolve. Alternatively, they can be added to water, allowed to dissolve and the water sipped.

As with the homeopathic remedies suggested in this guide, because we are focused on protocols and programs you simply need to administer the tissue salts noted in the manner described.

If you were to use the remedies for first aid or general home remedies during acute ailments or as supplementation, then the process is different. A general guideline would be:

Dosage varies according to the situation. Unless otherwise stipulated or prescribed the general rule of thumb is that for chronic cases, 2-4 pillules can be taken at least twice daily and up to four times daily. In acute conditions, take 2-4 pillules every hour or two. During intense situations they can be taken every 10-15 minutes.

What are Bach Flower Remedies?

Dr Edward Bach, a former Harley Street physician, discovered 38 remedies that coincide with specific mental and emotional states. 37 of these are based on single wild flowers and tree blossoms found in the English countryside. They are made by infusing spring water with the wild flowers and tree blossoms, either by means of the sun-steeped method or by boiling. The final essence, Rock Water, is made from the water of a natural spring with healing properties.

The most well-known of the Bach Flower Essences is Rescue Remedy or Five Flower Remedy. It is in fact a blend of 5 of the single Bach Flower Remedies.

The flower remedies treat the individual, not the disease or symptoms of the disease, by working specifically on their emotional state. Negative attitudes are transformed into optimism and the body's innate ability to self-heal is encouraged.

Dosage

Bach Flower Remedies can be administered by adding 2 drops of the selected remedy or remedies to a cup of water and sipping at intervals.

Alternatively, add 2 drops of each chosen remedy to a 30ml bottle of mineral water. From this take 4 drops 4 times daily until relief is experienced.

The mother tinctures contain alcohol as a preservative. If you are unable to ingest alcohol or uncomfortable doing so, simply add the essences to hot water and leave for a few minutes. The alcohol will evaporate.

HOMEOPROPHYLAXIS – A NATURAL ALTERNATIVE TO VACCINATION

Homeoprophylaxis is not a substitute for vaccines. They do not contain the ingredients nor the additives of normal vaccines and don't force the production of antibodies.

Instead it is a homeopathic protocol which uses nosodes to stimulate an appropriate immune response to natural disease. Very simply put the immune system is stimulated to learn how to get sick AND then how to heal the body.

Nosodes are very specific homeopathic remedies that are prepared from disease germs. However, none of germ remains in the final product. In essence, the pure disease energy is being administered which then stimulates the body's vital force.

Homeoprophylaxis is suitable for all children regardless of whether they have been fully or partially vaccinated or not been vaccinated at all. The only difference when following the protocol is that children who have been partially or fully vaccinated should ideally receive constitutional homeopathic treatment prior to beginning the program. The reason for this is that vaccinations will have altered their immune response. Constitutional treatment will balance the immune system to ensure that it responds to the homeoprophylaxis appropriately to ensure optimum benefit.

There are several Homeoprophylactic programs available. The one that will be outlined below is known as the Isaac Golden Program.

The following diseases are covered by the nosode mentioned in bold:
- Whooping Cough - **Pertussin**
- Pneumococcal Disease - **Pneumococcinum**
- Polio - **Lathyrus Sativa**
- Hib Influenza type B - **Haemophilus**
- Meningococcal Disease - **Meningococcinum**
- Tetanus - **Tetanus Toxin**
- Mumps - **Parotidinum**
- Measles - **Morbillinum**

The following diseases are not covered by the protocol:
- Hepatitis A or B
- Chickenpox
- Rotovirus
- Influenze

However, these nosodes can be added if necessary or desired.

The Isaac Golden Homoeoprophylaxis Program

Age to be given	Remedy	Doses	Potency
Year ONE			
1 month	Pertussin	1	200c
2 months	Pertussin	1 dose daily for 3 days	200c
4 months	Lathyrus Sativus	1	200c
5 months	Lathyrus Sativus	1	200c
6 months	Haemophilis	1	200c
7 months	Haemophilis Lathyrus Sativus	1 dose of each daily for 3 days	200c
9 months	Diptherinum	1	200c
10 months	Diptherinum	1 dose daily for 3 days	200c
11 months	Tetanus Toxin	1	200c
12 months	Tetanus Toxin	1 dose daily for 3 days	200c
Year TWO			
13 months	Pertussin	1 dose daily for 3 days	200c
14 months	Morbillinum	1	200c
15 months	Morbillinum	1 dose daily for 3 days	200c
16 months	Lathyrus Sativus	1 dose daily for 3 days	200c
17 months	Haemophilus	1 dose daily for 3 days	200c
19 months	Parotidinum	1	200c
20 months	Parotidinum	1 dose daily for 3 days	200c
22 months	Diptherinum	1 dose daily for 3 days	200c
24 months	Tetanus Toxin	1 dose daily for 3 days	200c

Year THREE			
26 months	Lathyrus Sativus	1	200c
28 months	Haemophilus	1 dose daily for 3 days	200c
32 months	Pertussin	1 dose daily for 3 days	200c
Year FOUR			
41 months	Tetanus Toxin	1 dose daily for 3 days	200c
46 months	Haemophilis	1 dose daily for 3 days	200c
Year FIVE			
50 months	Diptherinum	1 dose daily for 3 days	200c
54 months	Morbillinum	1 dose daily for 3 days	200c
56 months	Lathyrus Sativus	1 dose daily for 3 days	200c
60 months	Tetanus Toxin	1 dose daily for 3 days	200c

Prophylactic Remedies

The word prophylactic comes from the Greek term meaning "an advance guard". This is such an apt description as medically the word refers to a preventative measure, more specifically a medication, remedy or treatment that is used to fight off and prevent a disease from occurring.

Nosodes (as typically used in the Isaac Golden Program) can be difficult to find. A prophylactic remedy can then be used instead and will serve the same purpose.

There is usually more than one prophylactic remedy that can be substituted. If you find that you need to use a prophylactic, simply refer to the table below to make an appropriate selection.

It also notes prophylactics for diseases that are not covered by the Isaac Golden Program. These may be particularly useful when travelling to areas where there is a greater risk of contracting a disease such as Cholera, Diptheria or Rabies, and in instances where you feel it is appropriate to prevent or minimise the risk of contracting a specific disease such as Chicken Pox.

Nosode	Disease	Prophylactic	Dose	Potency
Varicellinum	Chicken Pox	Antimonium Tart Pulsatilla Rhus Tox	1 dose daily for 3 days	200c
Choleratoxinum	Cholera	Arsenicum Alb Cuprum Ac Veratrum Alb	1 dose daily for 3 days	200c
Diptherinum; Pyrogenium	Diptheria	Apis Mercurias Cyan	1 dose daily for 3 days	200c
Hydrophobinum	Rabies	Lyssinum Stramonium	1 dose daily for 3 days	200c
Morbillinum	Measles	Aconitum Nap Arsenicum Alb Pulsatilla	1 dose daily for 3 days	200c
Parotidinum	Mumps	Pilcarpine Trifolium Rep	1 dose daily for 3 days	200c
Pertussinum	Whooping Cough	Cuprum Met Drosera Vaccinum	1 dose daily for 3 days	200c
Polio (Mixed Nosode)	Polio	Carbolic Ac Lathyrus Sativus Physostigma Polio (Salk)	1 dose daily for 3 days	200c
Rubella Nosode	German Measles	Pulsatilla	1 dose daily for 3 days	200c
Variolinum	Small Pox	Antimonium Tart Hydrastis Kali Cyan	1 dose daily for 3 days	200c
Tetanotoxinum	Tetanus	Ledum Pal Thuja	1 dose daily for 3 days	200c

Supplementary Protection Program

Nosodes can be given as a booster at any time and is especially useful during an outbreak. The remedies indicated below can be used alongside the Homeoprophylaxis Program to further strengthen the immune system and to provide additional protection following definite exposure to an infection.

- **Chicken Pox**
  Varicella 30c once daily for 7 days during an outbreak.
- **Diptheria**
  Diptherinum 200c weekly for 4-6 weeks during an outbreak OR
  Diptherinum 30c once daily for 7 days.
- **Glandular Fever**
  Glandular Fever Nosode 30c once daily for 7 days during an outbreak.
- **Haemophilia**
  Haemophilis 1M every 2 weeks during a Hib outbreak.
- **Influenza and Colds**
  One dose of **Psorinum 200c** in Autumn will strengthen the immune system against the cold and flu viruses.
  Influenzinum et Baccilinum 200c every 3-4 weeks during the flu season will provide further protection.
  Oscillococcinum 200c twice daily for 7 days at the first sign of a cold or flu will shorten the duration.
- **Measles**
  Morbillinum 200c weekly for 3 weeks during an outbreak. OR
  Morbillinum 30c once daily for 7 days.
- **Mumps**
  Parotidinum 200c weekly during an epidemic or following contact with a carrier OR
  Parotidinum 30c once daily for 7 days.
- **Polio**
  Polio Mix 30c once daily for 7 days during an outbreak.
- **Rubella**
  In this instance acquiring natural immunity is best. Therefore, the ideal is therefore to allow an otherwise healthy child to acquire a mild bout of German Measles.
  However, if protection is required then use either **Rubella Nosode 200c** or **Pulsatilla 30c** twice a week for 2 weeks during an outbreak or following contact with a carrier.

- **Scarlet Fever**
  Scarletinum 30c once daily for 7 days during an outbreak.
- **Tetanus**
  Ledum Palustre 30c, 3 doses daily for 3 days following breakage of the skin.
- **Tonsillitus/Quinsy**
  A dose of **Barita Carbonica 30c** at the very first sign of inflammation can stop it progressing.
- **Whooping Cough**
  Pertussin 200c twice weekly for 3 weeks following contact with a carrier OR
  Pertussin 30c once daily for 7 days during an outbreak.

SIDE-EFFECTS OF VACCINATIONS

As previously mentioned there is a wealth of information available outlining the pros and cons of vaccinating and of course much has been written about the risks associated with vaccinating. Therefore, the potential side-effects are merely noted here with no further elaboration.

This is merely to provide a general awareness. It is always useful to have an inkling of how your little one may respond, particularly in the short-term, if you do choose to vaccinate. This allows you to be prepared and to have remedies on hand for the less severe reactions such as irritability, fever, runny nose etc.

Potential Short-term Side-effects

- Skin reactions
- Fever
- Vomiting, diarrhoea
- Cough, runny nose, ear infection
- High-pitched screaming, persistent crying
- Collapse or shock-like episodes
- Excessive sleepiness
- Seizure disorders - convulsions, epilepsy
- Infantile spasms
- Loss of muscle control
- Inflammation of the brain
- Blood disorders - Thrombocytopenia, Haemolytic Anaemia
- Diabetes and Hypoglycaemia
- Death and SIDS

Potential Long-term Side-effects

- Severe neurological damage
- Brain damage
- Learning disabilities

- Hyperactivity
- Allergy and hypersensitivity
- General damage to the immune system
- Slow viruses
- Genetic abnormalities e.g. "Jumping Gene" phenomenon
- Viral transference
- Trigger mechanism for immune system diseases
- Dynamic (miasmatic) changes

MINIMISING VACCINATION SIDE-EFFECTS

If you've decided to vaccinate or partially vaccinate your little one there will always be a risk of reaction to the immunisation. At the very least it's a shock to their little system, not only physically but mentally and emotionally as well.

It's instinctive for a parent to want to minimise their pain and discomfort as well as deal with any potential side-effects and risks.

An easy to follow guide is set out below which will do just that. It will enable you to support your baby mentally and emotionally as well as physically by minimising the risks associated with vaccinating and also reducing potential side-effects and reactions that may occur.

Mental and Emotional Support

Bach Flower Remedies are incredibly effective yet gentle enough to be used on newborns. The obvious one to reach for prior to the appointment as well as after is **Rescue Remedy** which is a blend of 5 individual Bach Flower Remedies. It contains Impatiens, Star of Bethlehem, Cherry Plum, Rock Rose and Clematis. A few drops diluted in water, juice or even their milk bottle will help to calm baby and restore a sense of security.

Physical Support

Vitamin C (Calcium Ascorbate) strengthens the immune system to fight off toxins and infections. Specific to vaccinating, it has been shown to greatly reduce the risk of SIDS as well as respiratory distress following immunisations.

It should be given for 1 week prior to vaccinating and continued for 7-21 days after vaccinating.

The guideline regarding dosage is 100gr per month of age.

- Infants up to age 2:   100gr to 250gr per day
- Ages 2 to 5:   250gr to 500gr per day
- Ages 5 and up: 500gr to 1gr per day

Holistic Support using Homeopathy

A Homeopathic pre- and post-vaccination protocol can support your little one physically, mentally and emotionally through the process of vaccination.

Homeopathy is perfectly safe to be taken by newborns and can be purchased in powder form which can simply be rubbed on their gums. This is particularly useful if they are being exclusively breastfed and not yet drinking from a bottle or still too young to take a pillule.

If they are drinking independently but refuse the pillule, it can be diluted in their bottle or cup of water, juice or even milk.

- **Ledum 30c**
  1 dose 1 hour prior to vaccination.
  1 dose every 12 hours for 1 day thereafter.
  This will help to reduce any swelling, redness and inflammation as a result of the vaccination. It also reduces the risk of infection and promotes healing of the puncture wound.

- **Arnica 30c**
  1 dose 1 hour prior to vaccination.
  1 dose every 8 hours for 2 days thereafter.
  This will help to reduce any long-term consequences associated with the trauma of vaccinating as well as reduce any associated pain, swelling, inflammation and bruising. It will also encourage more rapid healing.

- **Aconite 30c**
  2 doses daily for 3 days following the vaccination.
  This will alleviate any shock, fright, anxiety and fear as a result of being vaccinated and help to restore a sense of calm and security.

- **Thuja 30c**
  1 dose every 8 hours for 3 days following the vaccination.
  This remedy has been found to reduce the bad effects of vaccines and to alleviate associated side-effects. It encourages elimination of toxins introduced by the vaccination and restoration of balance.

- **Chamomilla 30c**
  Use if niggly, crying and upset, craving consolation and comfort.
  1 dose every 20 minutes until symptoms subside up to a maximum of 5 doses.
- **Belladonna 30c**
  Use if a fever develops.
  1 dose every 10-15 minutes until fever subsides or up to a maximum of 5 doses.

Isopathic Treatment

Another option is to make use of Isopathic Treatment which refers to using the potentised vaccine, also known as the homeopathic antidote. It is made by using the actual vaccine and producing a homoeopathically potentised form thereof.

A homeopathic antidote is therefore available for every single conventional vaccine used e.g. there is a Varicella (Chicken Pox) antidote, MMR antidote, Hep B antidote, even a Vitamin K antidote.

The Potentised Vaccine/Antidote Protocol is very easy to follow:
- 2 days before the vaccination, give the **potentised vaccine** e.g. DKTP in **200c** potency.
- **Thuja 30c** can be given alongside this - 2 doses 12 hours apart.
- 1 dose of the **potentised vaccine** in **200c** potency, immediately after having the vaccination done.

If symptoms do develop it is a healing crisis or disease mimic. The **actual nosode** should then be given to shorten the duration and ease discomfort. Give 2 doses in either **30c or 200c** potency 8 hours apart.

An example would be where you use the potentised vaccine of Diptheria as described above and after being vaccinated your little one begins to show symptoms. You should then give the Diptheria Nosode, Diptherinum in either 30c or 200c potency.

If no further vaccinations are to be given in the near future, then the potentised vaccine should be given one month later in ascending potencies over a period of 4 consecutive days.
In other words:

- Day 1: Potentised vaccine in 30c
- Day 2: Potentised vaccine in 200c
- Day 3: Potentised vaccine in 1M
- Day 4: Potentised vaccine in 10M

This will help to correct any possible disturbances from the vaccination to the deeper energy levels and constitution.

If complications do still occur after following the Potentised Vaccine Protocol, then the potentised vaccine in 200c potency should be dissolved in water and taken over a period of 3 days.

It is VERY important to remember that potentised vaccines do NOT confer immunity nor do they treat disease. This protocol does not serve as an alternative to vaccinations. Its purpose is to minimise the side-effects of having vaccinations.

VACCINATION DETOX PROGRAMS

Vaccinations will inevitably introduce specific toxins into the body. These will place added stress on particular pathways and organs of the body. Eliminating these toxins as gently as possible will reduce the stress and strengthen the affected body systems and organs, encouraging them to return to optimal health and functioning.

The detox options below can be followed any time after having a vaccination or course of vaccinations done. All are very gentle and safe while encouraging healthy elimination of any toxins introduced.

Homeopathic Vaccination Detox

A gentle detox that takes place over a two-week period and is perfectly safe for infants:

- **Day 1-3**
  Thuja 30c
  1 dose every 8 hours for 3 days.
  This will encourage elimination of all toxins introduced by the vaccine.
- **Day 4-6**
  Silica 30c
  1 doses every 8 hours for 3 days.
  This will draw toxins out of the tissues and into the blood stream for elimination.
- **Day 7-13**
  Mercurius Solubilis 30c
  1 dose every 8 hours for a period of 1 week.
  This is especially useful where the vaccine contains mercury or traces of mercury (and/or aluminium or other metals). It encourages safe elimination of these toxins.
- **Day 14**
  Homeopathathic Antidote 200c
  1 dose.
  This will calm the discomfort and after effects specific to the vaccination that has been administered.

Tissue Salt Vaccination Detox

An easy to follow, gentle detox that takes place over a one-month period. As with the homeopathic detox it is perfectly safe for infants:

- **Calc Sulph (Tissue Salt Number 3)**
  This will encourage detoxification of the liver.
- **Kali Sulph (Tissue Salt Number 7)**
  This encourages general detoxification and strengthens the respiratory system.
- **Nat Phos (Tissue Salt Number 10)**
  This encourages general detoxification, addresses acidity imbalance and strengthens the digestive system.
- **Nat Sulph (Tissue Salt Number 11)**
  This has general anti-inflammatory properties, encourages detoxification of the liver and strengthens the respiratory system.
- **Silicea (Tissue Salt Number 12)**
  This is known as the homeopathic purger or cleanser. It encourages elimination of toxins and any foreign objects from the body. In addition, it helps to improve skin and bone health.

Simply add 3 tablets of each Tissue Salt to 250ml-500ml water and sip throughout the day. It can of course be added to the bottle of infants. For those not yet drinking from a bottle or cup e.g. still being exclusively breastfed, the tablets can be crushed into a fine powder and rubbed on the gums.

Do this daily for a period of one month.

Detox Bath

A calming and detoxifying bath is easy to prepare. Simply add the following to warm bath water and soak for 20-30 minutes. Alternatively, add to a foot bath and soak feet for 20-30 minutes.

- ½ cup **Bentonite Clay**
- ½ cup **Epsom Salts**
- 3 drops **Coriander Essential Oil**
- 3 drops **Geranium Essential Oil**
- 3 drops **Frankincense Essential Oil**
- 3 drops **Helichrysum Essential Oil**

The Tissue Salts mentioned above can also be added, 2-3 tablets of each:
- **Calc Sulph (Tissue Salt Number 3)**
- **Kali Sulph (Tissue Salt Number 7)**
- **Nat Phos (Tissue Salt Number 10)**
- **Nat Sulph (Tissue Salt Number 11)**
- **Silicea (Tissue Salt Number 12)**

This is suitable for little ones from 6 months of age. If under 6 months leave out the Essential Oils.

Vaccination Support Kit Shopping List

- Vitamin C (Calcium Ascorbate) Powder
- Homeopathic Remedies
  Aconite 30c
  Arnica 30c
  Belladonna 30c
  Chamomilla 30c
  Ledum 30c
  Thuja 30c
  Potentised Vaccine 30c, 200c, 1M and 10M
  Vaccine Nosode 200c
- Biochemical Tissue Salts
  Calc Sulph (Number 3)
  Kali Sulph (Number 7)
  Nat Phos (Number 10)
  Nat Sulph (Number 11)
  Silicea (Number 12)
- Bentonite Clay
- Epsom Salts
- Essential Oils
  Coriander
  Geranium
  Frankincense
  Helichrysum

BIBLIOGRAPHY

An Introduction & Guide to Flower Remedies
The 38 Flower Remedies

Desktop Guide to Keynotes and Confirmatory Symptoms
Roger Morrison, M.D.

Fundamentals of Acute Homoeopathic Prescribing
Yves Roire and Paul Callinan

Homoeopathic Alternatives to Immunisation
A guide for travellers and parents looking for an alternative to being immunised.
Susan Curtis

Pocket Manual of Homoeopathic Materia Medica and Repertory
William Boericke, M.D.

Schussler's Twelve Tissue Remedies
William Boericke and W.A. Dewey

The Complete Practitioner's Manual of Homoeoprophylaxis
A Practical Handbook of Homeopathic Immunisation
Dr Isaac Golden

Vaccination
A Guide for Making Personal Choices
Dr Hans -Peter Studer

Vaccine Free: Homeopathic Education for the Immune System
Kate Birch

ABOUT THE AUTHOR

Dorae Smith originally studied law and spent many years working in the legal and corporate field.

In 2007, while living and working in the UK she decided to follow her passion for natural medicine. She retrained as a Naturopath, specialising in Homeopathy and spent over a decade in private practice in the UK before returning home to South Africa.

After the birth of her baby girl in 2016 she inevitably began making all-natural products at home for her little one.

This sparked her interest in product development. She wanted to create all-natural, gentle products with purpose. And not only for little ones but for everyone.

In 2018 she turned her focus to caring for her little girl and creating an all-natural product range. And so bubiroo came about - a range of all-natural, preservative free, gentle yet therapeutic products handmade with love by a Naturopath mama.

She currently lives in Port Elizabeth, South Africa. When time allows, she writes children's stories and of course books relating to natural medicine.

This book came about due to often being asked about vaccinations while in practice and of course having to make the very personal choice of whether to vaccinate or not when her little girl came along.

www.ingramcontent.com/pod-product-compliance
Lightning Source LLC
Chambersburg PA
CBHW031512210526
45463CB00008B/3205